Living on a pra roller coaster ride that almost five months while in the Neonatal Intensive Care Unit. We had hit rock bottom and the only thing we could do was live our life on prayer. We struggled with our faith from time to time and then with the power of prayer, witnessed miracles in front of our very own eyes. Our faith became stronger and our little girl eventually started to get better. We were grieving for our baby boy that was also our little girl's twin; he had passed away 36 hours after birth. It was a daily struggle trying to keep our heads above water as we feared we would lose her too. I'm hoping that sharing our story will help other parents going through a similar situation and give them hope. Life is all about choices and how we choose to handle the situations that are thrown at us. Some things in life we have no control over and we just have to have faith that things will be okay.

"I remember staring at an incubator from across the room for many hours, weeks and months, wanting to touch and hold her but knowing at that moment I couldn't. I feared for her life every minute of every day. I watched as her condition got worse and life support was increased. I watched doctors rush in and out from time to time trying to save our fragile little girl that was barely clinging onto life. She was born fighting. Fighting for her life, fighting to prove doctors wrong and fighting for us. It's almost like she knows we can't do this without her. We can't lose her too."- Tiffani Elmgren

Table of Contents:

About the Author	Page....4
My Nightmare	Page....8
22 Weeks & 1 Day	Page....13
Delivery	Page....18
The Nightmare Cont'd	Page....22
Teddy	Page....40
The Power of Prayer	Page....44
Home for the Holidays?	Page....51
A New Year	Page....57
A New Beginning	Page....67
Insights	Page....71

A little about me,

I grew up in a small town in Wisconsin with just over 600 people. We didn't have a lot of money or have the finer things in life but we had each other. We were part of a community where everyone helped each other out. I spent a lot of time with my great-grandmother whom was very involved with our church. She cleaned the church, kept up the flowers & plants and served her lord. I looked up to her and tried my hardest to follow in her footsteps. My fondest memories were always walking the 2 miles to church with her every Sunday. My grandmother never had a driver's license, so she walked most places; or rode the school bus when she volunteered at our school. She was the most selfless person I had known and would help anyone in need.

When I was 16, I was so excited to get my driver's license because then I could drive my grandma around so she wouldn't have to walk. She was in her seventies and probably one of the fittest grandmas in our town. Shortly after that, she was diagnosed with cancer and lost her battle after only six months. She became very sick and it broke my heart to watch her suffer. It was even harder on me because she passed away exactly two months after my father had. I was in Texas when I got the phone call that my grandma had passed away and I was so angry at myself for not being there for her. I was with my dad's side of the family; my dad had committed suicide and it was a messy situation and I felt it was best to be in the comfort of my family that was closest to him. I had lost my two best friends that summer.

I wasn't very popular in high school but I did have a group of close knit friends; mostly guys. I was kind of a tom boy and just got along better with the guys; although I did have girlfriends too. My sophomore year of high school, I met my high school sweetheart. We spent most of our time together when we weren't in school or working. We had the best of both worlds because we were also best friends. After 5 years of dating, he asked me to marry him and we are still going strong today. I didn't think I could love him anymore than I did on our wedding day; until we went through our worst nightmare together. That is when I realized how much he held me together when I was falling apart.

I am a new first time mom to my surviving 23 week twin. She had a very rough start to life but has taught us so much about strength, courage, faith and the power of prayer. My husband and I have been home from the NICU for 4 months now. We spent 136 days at Children's Hospital in St. Paul, MN with our daughter. We were terrified coming home with all of the medical equipment and medications that she needed to survive. I resigned my full time job at our local hospital to become a stay at home mom. I knew in my heart this was the best decision for our family; our daughter needed me and quite frankly I was in no shape to go back to work after everything we had just went through. The things we went through no parent should have to go through, but so many do and I want to make awareness of that. I'm hoping that sharing my story will bring comfort and hope to other parents going through a similar situation. My story may have "triggers" for parents that have already been through the NICU; so please read with caution. I want our story to give others hope that miracles do happen and to never give up despite what tries to knock you down. With the power of prayer, I have watched miracles happen in front of my very own eyes.

My Nightmare

August 31st, 2017-

  I woke up this morning feeling good. It was the first morning in a of couple weeks that I didn't have morning sickness. I kissed my husband goodbye and got ready for my day at work. Today is my husband's birthday so I was thinking of all the possible ways I could make it special for him. I felt like he deserved the "Husband of the Year" award for constantly doting on me the last four months. He wouldn't let me do laundry because that would entail me carrying laundry baskets down two flights of stairs and he would not have that while I was carrying his babies. He was so excited to be a daddy and took on a lot of the household chores. I was extremely fatigued and sick since very early on in my pregnancy. We joked that we didn't understand why they called it "Morning Sickness" because I had it all day long, almost every day. I couldn't keep food down and after work I would come home and go straight to bed; but I wouldn't change one second of that if I could go back in time.

  About halfway through my work day I started having pain in my ribs. I brushed it off and figured it was nothing. I often worried about unnecessary things because of my anxiety and figured this was just one of those times. A couple of hours had passed by and I was still having pains. I began to panic thinking of all the things that could possibly go wrong. Being that I work for the hospital, I went to one of my nurse co-workers and asked for their opinion. After a few minutes, they had advised that I go to the OB unit to have things checked out to make sure everything was okay. When I got to OB, they put the monitors on me and I could immediately hear both of my babies. I took a breath of relief. All of my vitals looked good and they could pick up both of my babies' heart beats on the monitor. They didn't want to take any chances though, so advised me to wait until my OB doctor could come in and check on me first. She was in another delivery but the nurses assured me she would be in as soon as she could.

Shortly after that, my husband had arrived. I had called him at work and asked him to come. As we waited for my doctor to come, we could hear both of our babies on the monitor and I could feel them kicking up a storm. At that point we weren't very concerned and thought that I just needed the all clear from my doctor and then we could go home.

After several of hours, a different doctor became available so she came to check on me instead. After only a short few seconds of her checking my cervix, she got up and walked out of the room. Panic began to set in as we were wondering what was going on. She came right back in and stated that she had just paged a helicopter to come and airlift me to a different hospital. I began to cry as I was terrified of what was going on. She explained that I had ruptured membranes and I needed to get down to the specialists right away. I looked over at my husband and he was as white as a ghost. I told him to call his mother as I knew they wouldn't allow him in the helicopter with me. While he went to call his mom, the helicopter had shown up. My husband leaned over and gave me a kiss and stated that he would meet me at the other hospital as soon as he could get there.

The helicopter ride was one of the scariest rides of my life. I was terrified to what was happening and was afraid of losing my babies. The medics on the helicopter were very comforting and during the very short ride, they had put the monitors on me twice to check my babies.

I arrived at the other hospital within 15 minutes and was immediately hooked up to an ultrasound. After about an hour, my husband and his parents had arrived. We were all terrified as we waited for any kind of answers. One of the doctors had come in and explained that I had ruptured membranes and was on strict bed rest until I delivered. I was only 22 weeks pregnant and had just found out two weeks prior that I was having one boy and one girl. We were so excited and now we are living our worst nightmare. The doctors didn't have an answer to why my membranes had ruptured but we knew the clock was ticking and we didn't have much time before our babies would arrive.

In the meantime, many doctors, nurses, social workers and chaplains had been in and out of my room; but I distinctly remember the doctor that came in from the NICU to explain to my husband and I what the NICU would look like "if" our babies would survive. That's when things really started to hit me. We could lose both of our babies. How could this be happening to us? What did I do wrong? The guilt was setting in and I had never been more terrified in my life.

The doctor explained that they didn't consider babies viable until 23 weeks gestation and that they wouldn't intervene if I delivered before 23 weeks. He also stated that having a baby that premature would more than likely lead to many disabilities if they survived at all and explained that we could terminate my pregnancy if we wished. My heart sank into the pit of my stomach. I was emotional and frightened and then I became angry. What do you mean "you wouldn't intervene if they came before then?" How could you not try to save my babies? Terminating my pregnancy had never crossed my mind and it was not an option. There was no way we were giving up on our babies no matter what the outcome may be.

After the doctor had left, my husband kissed me and said everything would be okay. I could tell he was just as afraid as I was but he was trying to keep me calm. We always tried to find the silver lining in life, but this time it was hard for me. How could I live without my babies? I kept telling myself this had to be a nightmare; this really couldn't be happening. We had tried for two years to get pregnant; why would God do this to us? My faith was strong and I had always served my lord to the best of my ability, so why would he do this to me?

Soon after that, survival mode kicked in. I was determined that my babies weren't coming out and we would make it a lot farther in this pregnancy. I was going to do everything in my power to give my babies a fighting chance.

22 Weeks & 1 Day

The next morning I got up to use the restroom. As soon as I sat down I could feel something bulging out of my cervix and I knew something was wrong. I carefully stood up and waddled to the bathroom door. My mother-in-law could see the panic on my face and immediately called for a nurse. They carefully got me back into bed and I was quickly surrounded by doctors. My baby girl's placenta; still intact, was on the outside of my cervix. The doctors were astonished that it had not ruptured and I wasn't having contractions. They quickly rushed me to emergency delivery.

I remember lying on my bed in the middle of the hall as all of the doctors and nurses around me quickly discussed on what the next plan of action would be being that I was only 22 weeks and 1 day pregnant. I cried as I remembered what the NICU doctor had told me about not intervening to save them until 23 weeks gestation. I begged them to do whatever it took to help my babies survive.

I cried as I laid there feeling like I had no control over what was going to happen and that I was going to lose both of my babies. After the team was done talking, one of the doctors came up and bent over my bed. She told me, "You are going to have to push and let mother nature take its course." I balled as I told her I couldn't. I wasn't giving up on my babies and I was determined to make it further along. If I pushed that would mean my babies would die. I told the doctor that I was not ready to push and that I wouldn't do it. I could tell she was frustrated with how stubborn I was being, and I understood that they were concerned about my safety also but my babies were my only priority.

My husband held my hand as the nurses rolled me back into my room. They put me in the Trendelenburg position to see if gravity would guide my baby girl's placenta back into my cervix. The Trendelenburg position is where you are tilted so your feet are higher than your head. Remarkably it worked! My baby girl's placenta had gone back into my cervix and the doctors were amazed. They put me back on strict orders that I could not get out of bed at all as gravity could undo what had just happened. I didn't care if I had to lie in bed until I was nine months pregnant; if that's what it would take then that is what I would do.

The next couple of days I stayed in bed and didn't get up once. Nothing had changed so my doctor agreed to let me get up to use the bathroom so I could have a break from my bedpan. I went into the bathroom and sat down and could immediately feel my baby girl's placenta starting to bulge back out. I screamed for the nurse that was right outside my bathroom door. She came in and had gently moved me back into my bed.

I had made my intentions clear a few days prior that I would not be pushing my babies out at this point, so the nurse put me back into bed and called the doctor to let them know what had happened. They tried putting me back in the Trendelenburg position again to see if that would work again, but after several hours it didn't seem to be working.

The doctor put me on the ultrasound and explained that my cervix had been dilated just enough for my baby girl's placenta to bulge out and that it had closed again so the part of the placenta that was bulging out would not be able to go back in. My baby girl was still inside her placenta on the inside of my cervix but part of the placenta had leaked out and now wouldn't be able to go back in. He ordered strict bed rest again with no getting out of bed. Any sort of gravity could end my pregnancy.

A few more days went by and the part of the placenta that was on the outside of my cervix kept getting bigger. Cervical fluid was leaking from the side the baby was on to the part of the placenta that was bulging out; so that meant her side of the placenta was getting smaller and smaller with less cervical fluid which was vital for her survival. We were almost at the 23 week gestation mark. I needed to make it to at least 23 weeks if I wanted any chance at my babies surviving.

At midnight that night I had become 23 weeks pregnant which meant that if I now delivered; my babies would have a fighting chance. The nurses immediately started me on a magnesium drip which would help the brain development of my babies. The side effects were miserable but I was so focused on my babies' survival that it didn't matter how much pain or discomfort I had to go through; I would do it. They also gave me two doses of steroids to help their lung development. Babies' lungs don't usually mature until 36 weeks gestation and are one of the last organs to develop. Obviously, no parent wants to deliver their baby prematurely but we had a slight relief knowing we had made it to the 23 week mark. Now our next goal was to make it farther.

As the next few days went by, my placenta kept leaking cervical fluid and kept increasing in size outside of my cervix. I don't remember much in those few days except I was in a lot of pain. I had lost all my dignity as I had to go to the bathroom on a pad in my bed. I could no longer use a bed pan because we were afraid that it would tear my placenta open if it got snagged. My baby girl's placenta was now the size of a grapefruit lying outside of my cervix on my bed. I could barely move those few days because I feared my placenta would burst and my baby girl would die.

Later on during that day, the doctor came in and told me that my daily blood work results had come back and that I had become septic. He stated I needed to deliver as soon as possible for the best possible outcome for both myself and my babies. I cried because I felt as if my body had failed me. I would have lied there for months just to keep my babies safe and now that was no longer a possibility because my placenta that had been bulging out for days had become infected and was making my babies and I sick. The doctor told me that they would be giving me a medication to speed up my contractions that I was now having and that I would be delivering my babies that day.

It was only a couple of hours before I was really feeling my contractions and my doctor said it was time if I wanted an epidural. My doctor called for anesthesia to come and they had to administer the epidural with me lying on my side which had never been done before at that hospital. I could not sit up and do it the usual way because that could have also ruptured my placenta.

My doctor returned to my room to check my cervix and stated that I was dilated to 5-6 centimeters. He explained that I didn't need to be completely dilated all of the way because my babies were so small and that it was time for delivery. At that moment my family and I prayed like we have never prayed before. Our church, family, friends, community and people we didn't even know were praying for us and our babies. This is the moment I realized the power of prayer and how it brings so many people together.

Delivery

The nurses wheeled my bed into the delivery room that was connected to a resuscitation room. My husband was at my bedside and I could see the fear on his face also. Our families were out in the waiting room making phone calls and asking people to pray. I begged the lord to keep my babies safe and let them be okay. The doctor had told me that as soon as my babies had arrived, they would be immediately taken to the resuscitation room so I wouldn't be able to get more than a quick glance at them. He told me that he admired my determination and love for my babies. It had been ten days since this had all started and I had made it to 23 weeks and 3 days. Within that time frame was the difference of whether or not doctors could intervene and try to help or not.

I cried as I began to push. I was terrified at what the outcome would be. One short push and my baby girl had arrived. I caught a quick glimpse and couldn't believe how small she was. I watched as the nurses quickly whisked her back into the resuscitation room. I didn't know if she was alive or not and before I could even ask; the doctor had told me I needed to push again. Our baby boy arrived after two pushes and again was whisked away. My husband and I cried as we begged to know if they were okay. What seemed like an eternity went by and our doctor came back and told us both of our babies were currently on life support by alive. The smallest size breathing tubes that are made barely fit down their throats and into their lungs. We were unable to see them at that time but the doctor assured us that later that day we would be able to see them down in the NICU.

I was taken back to my room where we were reunited with our families. At that moment it became clear to us why the cut-off for viability was 23 weeks. My husband and I didn't understand this when we were first admitted, on why one week made a difference whether or not they would try to save our babies. It wasn't a matter of "if" they would try to save them; it was that in just one short week our babies had grown just enough for the smallest breathing tubes to barely fit into their lungs. If I would have delivered when I first arrived, there would have been no way the breathing tubes would have fit. We had continued to pray that our babies would be okay as we waited to meet them.

Later that day, we were taken down to the NICU. It was a whole different world down there; that most people can't imagine unless they have been through it or witnessed it. When we first walked in, we had to check in with the front desk and stop at the sanitizing wash station before entering through to the NICU. Once we got to our babies' rooms we were instructed to sanitize again every time we entered or left the room. Our babies were in incubators and in separate rooms. The rooms were dark and there were blankets draped over their incubators. The nurses explained that they try to mimic the womb with it being dark and quiet in the rooms. Loud noises and light are way too much stimulation for babies born that premature. We were advised to talk in slow whispers.

The first room we entered was our baby girl, Loretta June. She was in an incubator with a small cloth draped over her eyes. Her eyes were still fused shut and her skin was so thin it was transparent. There was so much equipment and monitors around her incubator. I peeked through the blanket to look in at her. I had never seen anything so small. My hand covered her entire 1lb 3oz body. It was intimidating seeing the breathing tubes and ventilators along with all the wires and leads but I had asked if I could touch her. The nurse had shown me how to gently place my finger in on her. I was afraid I would tear her skin because it was so thin. She explained not to use stroking motions while touching our babies because that is also too much stimulation. After a few moments of my finger pressed against her hand, I could feel her squeeze it. My heart melted and I became emotional as I felt that this was her way of telling me it would be okay. All five of the tips of her fingers barely covered the tip of my one finger.

After a few minutes, I quietly closed her incubator door and asked if I could see my son. Teddy was in the room next door. We walked in and he looked the same as our Loretta, only a little bigger. He was 1lb 8oz and also had all of the equipment and monitors on him. We quietly opened his incubator and again I placed my finger in his hand. He also had a cloth draped over his eyes that were fused shut. I felt so much love in my heart and thanked God for blessing me with two miracles. We had no idea what we were in for and we were so afraid but I knew we needed to be strong for our warriors. They literally had the fight of their lives.

The Nightmare Continues

The next day, the doctor approached my husband and I and asked if we had a moment to talk. She asked us to take a seat and explained that Teddy had a bilateral Grade 4 brain bleed and was not responding to blood pressure medications. His lungs weren't developed enough and even with the jet ventilator and steroids on board, he wasn't responding. She suggested we put him on the do not resuscitate and stated that even if he was able to survive this he would probably never see, hear, walk, talk, eat, or even breathe on his own. He would have no quality of life. Everything was in slow motion now. My son will have a life with zero quality and there is nothing I can do to help him. I'm going to lose my baby boy and I can't stop repeating that to myself in my head. I'm frozen..shaken..stuck. The doctor gave us three options; 1. Keep him on life support and live his life for him if he survives this, 2. Put him on DNR and if things get worse, let him go, Or 3. Withdraw care, give him morphine and let him pass on his own without any pain. It took us several hours to make our decision; #3. Withdraw care. I felt so guilty because I felt like we were giving up on our son. I didn't want to let him go but somehow, as much as my heart ached, it told me that is was what we needed to do. Keeping him around to live a life of pain and suffering would be so selfish of us. All we would be able to do is wait for the day that his heart or his brain couldn't fight anymore. Nobody wants to live in pain fearing which day would be their last. So that was our decision.

We made the hardest decision of our lives to have his breathing support removed. The doctors administered morphine so he wouldn't feel any pain and then placed my son in my arms as my husband and I sat on the couch holding him for dear life. I felt like my heart was going to stop. My chest hurts so badly and I have a tight stabbing pain from my anxiety. My head hurts from the on and off crying. My sweet innocent baby doesn't even know what's about to happen and that's the hardest part. After five hours of holding him, taking our first and last pictures and feeling that life wasn't worth living, we said goodbye. September 12th at 12:37am is when our angel took his last breath and got his shiny little angel wings. I feel as if time was frozen. Everything is in slow motion. I feel like I can't breathe and that I'm completely empty. Why? What did he do to deserve this? Why do we deserve this as parents? What parent deserves to hold their baby in their arms as they take their last breath? Who deserves the pain of having to comfort their baby, just waiting for him to die? Nobody. I wish that upon no one ever.

The image of him lying there lifelessly in my arms is what I see every time I close my eyes. The feeling of my heart dropping when I finally heard his heart stop beating, yeah that feeling seems permanent now. It doesn't go away. It's an ache I'll never in my lifetime be able to get rid of. It's a still feeling now. It's constant.

Every second of every day is a repeat of this heartache. My pain can't be put into words. It was the most emotionally confusing and painful moment of my life. I never got to hear my baby cry. Never got to feed my baby. Never got to dress my baby. My baby never got to wear clothes. I never heard my baby cough. Never heard him sneeze. He fought every hour, every minute and every second of his life and now I struggle with the decision I made. Was it the right decision? I didn't want him to suffer and I didn't want him in pain but how can I live with all of this guilt?

Then it hits me that my little girl is in the room next door, also fighting for her life. This nightmare isn't over. Is it going to happen again? Will I lose her too? I can't handle this pain again. How am I going to keep it together for her?

I walked into her room and felt like it was dejavu. She looks so much like her twin brother. She is even smaller and more fragile looking. I reach in and put my finger in her hand and she immediately squeezes my finger as if she's telling me "it's okay mommy." I burst into tears as I think about everything that has happened. I fought for 10 days in the hospital to give my babies a fighting chance at survival. Doctors prepared me for the worst and someway, somehow I delivered both of my babies alive.

I spent 36 hours with my son before he took his last breath and now I'm living in fear, afraid to get attached to my daughter because I don't want to go through this pain again. Is this a cruel joke? Why would God bless me with twins and then take one away from me? I was on an emotional roller coaster and knew it was nowhere near the end. Even with my faith as strong as it was, I questioned my lord's intentions. I was angry with him for taking my baby boy.

People would tell me that "everything happens for a reason" but that is not what I wanted to hear. There is no logical reason that any parent should have to go through this. No parent should ever have to deal with watching their baby die.

Eventually, my anger turned into determination that my baby girl would beat the odds. I put all of my focus on her and nothing else. I knew my baby boy lived on in her and eventually I would need to grieve for him; but for now I had to focus on her. She needed to make it through this.

Over the next couple of days we sat by Loretta's incubator side when we could. I still needed to go back to my post-partum room to be checked on and given more medications for my infection. It was so hard being in the post-partum unit. I could hear babies crying down the hall that were being comforted by their mommies. I cried because I couldn't comfort mine. I didn't even know when I would be able to hold my little girl or when she would let out her first cry. We had so many unknowns and doctors were unable to give us answers because they didn't want to give us any sense of false hope.

Once I was discharged, I pretty much lived in Loretta's NICU room. I prayed non-stop that she would survive all of this. Later that day, the nurse came in and asked me if I wanted to hold her. My heart and eyes lit up and I couldn't believe what I was hearing. She was three days old and I would be holding her for the first time. I undressed and put a gown on and the nurses called for a respiratory therapist to come and help move her. It took three nurses and a respiratory therapist to help me get her out of her incubator. I bent over her incubator and got my body as close to her as I could before picking her up; it was crucial to keep her warm while she was outside of the incubator because she couldn't manage her body temperature on her own yet. I carefully moved to my chair with her on my bare skinned chest and warm blankets draped over her body. The nurses moved cords and wires and the respiratory therapist held her breathing tube at her mouth to make sure it didn't shift or get pulled out. Once I sat down the nurses taped all of her wires and breathing tube to my chest so that way they wouldn't move. Even the slightest tug on her breathing tube could have dislodged it out of place. I sat as still as I possibly could. I was terrified and intimidated to bump anything but my heart was so full to feel her on my chest.

An amazing thing happened while I held her. Her oxygen needs and heart rate started going down. The nurse explained that my baby girl was calming down and was more relaxed on my chest. The warmth of my body and the sound of my heart beat was what she needed. This was the first time I felt like I could actually do something for my baby girl. I couldn't do much else at this time but I could hold her; so that's what I did. I would hold her for periods of 4-6 hours straight being still and careful not to move. Her eyes were still fused shut and she didn't make any sounds; but this is the therapy I needed right now. Holding her comforted me.

A few days later, I had a lot of pain in my lower abdomen. I tried to brush it off and ignore it because I wanted to focus all of my attention on Loretta but the pain was unbearable. When my husband returned back to the hospital from work I explained to him what I was feeling and we decided to go to the emergency room on the other side of the hospital. I had a bad infection and was told that they were re-admitting me. I panicked; they couldn't admit me, I needed to be there for my baby. They hooked me up to IV antibiotics and admitted me to the hospital. I cried as I lay in my hospital bed wanting to be near my daughter. I could see the fatigue on my husband's face as he tried to go to Loretta's room to stay informed and get updated on her and come back to my room and get the update on what was going on with me. I begged for the nurses to allow me to go and see my baby but per hospital protocol that wasn't allowed.

After I had decided I was going to discharge myself against medical advice, one of the case managers came in and we had come to an agreement that I could go down and be with Loretta as long as I came back so the nurses could check my vitals and administer more IV medications. I agreed, so I went and spent my time in Loretta's room with my husband and my IV pole. Every three hours my husband would wheel me in my wheelchair back up to my room and the nurses would take my vitals and give me more medications. We tried to find humor in it and joked that "every three hours, I had to go check in with my parole officers to get more meds." After two days of this, I was finally feeling better and discharged. I give those nurses a lot of credit, they were just trying to do their job and I wasn't making it easy on them, but nothing was going to stop me from being there for my baby.

On September 21st, 11 days after Loretta was born; she stopped urinating. They gave her Lasix to help her urinate and routinely did x-rays every 12 hours to watch her lungs. The routine x-rays were also done to make sure her breathing tube was still in the correct place and to monitor her chronic lung disease from being born prematurely. Loretta had come off of the bili-light and opened her eyes for the very first time! We cried with excitement that we could finally see her beautiful eyes. Being she was so little; her eyes didn't have color yet but the nurse reassured us that over time they would change. The doctor ordered an echocardiogram and head ultrasound to check her heart and brain. They did one when she was born and she had a small hole in her heart and a Right Grade 2 & Left Grade 3 Brain Bleed. They stated they would monitor the small hole in her heart to see if it would close on its own. The head ultrasound still showed blood on her brain but it didn't look like new blood so they believed it was from when she was born. The doctors had said hopefully over the next couple of months the blood would resolve and no action would need to be taken; but they would monitor her closely to make sure she didn't have any new bleeding or swelling on her brain.

The next day Loretta's tummy had a dusky looking color on the outside and looked bloated. The x-ray showed that her intestines were irritated. Doctors immediately ran blood cultures and started her on antibiotics to be proactive. They started doing x-rays every 6 hours to monitor her condition until her results came back. When the results came back it showed that she had Necrotizing Enterocolitis, also known as NEC. The tissues of her intestines were inflamed and if they developed a perforation it could make her very sick or even be life threatening. The doctor came in and stated that they were going to start her on an aggressive antibiotic to treat the NEC but in order to do that they would need to do a procedure. They had ran out of her tiny little veins to put IVs in and would need to do a broviac procedure which would put a central line through her chest cavity into one of the larger veins close to her heart. We were terrified; again afraid we were going to lose our baby girl. My husband and I told them to do whatever they needed to do. We had put all of our trust in these doctors and nurses.

The way these providers worked was amazing. Every morning they did "roundings" where the care team of doctors, nurses, pharmacists, dieticians and pulmonologists would get together and round on each of the babies in the NICU. Parents are allowed to be a part of these meetings when they are discussing your child; so every morning I would go. It was amazing to listen to them talk and how they knew every little detail on my baby girl. They talked back and forth with each other to make sure she was getting the correct doses of medications based on her tiny weight, made sure her blood gasses looked good which meant that she was oxygenating well on her ventilator, made sure she was getting enough nutrition and discussed any results or procedures that they felt needed to be done.

Loretta was on many medications and vitamins to help control her blood pressure, glucose, iron, Vitamin A & D, potassium and sodium. They gave her caffeine every day which was supposed to encourage her lungs to breathe. She also was on scheduled Morphine and Ativan to help relax her and keep her calm so she wouldn't fight her ventilator. We were so amazed by how advanced the medical field had become and so impressed with our care team. We completely trusted them with our baby girl and knew they were doing everything they could to help her.

The next morning they started preparing Loretta for her broviac procedure. They gave her a blood transfusion, Lasix to help her urinate and put a catheter in.

I was terrified as many doctors, nurses, respiratory therapists, surgeons and techs all entered her room. It took an army to move her in her incubator to the operating room. The respiratory therapist needed to reach their hand in and hold the breathing tube at the lips of her mouth so it didn't move while they rolled her down the hall. The surgery techs slowly rolled her incubator while the nurses followed close behind in baby steps moving her IV poles, ventilator and monitors; being very careful to stay close so the cords didn't pull on Loretta's fragile little body. I was a nervous wreck as they took her away; I prayed and prayed as I waited for her return.

About an hour later, the surgeon came into her room and stated the surgery went well. I had a sigh of relief. He explained that they gave her Fentanyl for pain and also a paralysis medication so that she wouldn't feel anything. He told me not to be alarmed if she didn't move much until the next day as the paralysis medication would take time to wear off. They also started her on an antifungal medication twice a week to help prevent infection while she had the broviac line in.

I was so relieved when they rolled her back into her room. I just wanted to hold her and comfort her but I knew that I would not be able to do so that day, so I sat by her side reaching my hand through her incubator door. I wanted her to know, to feel, that I was there.

Over the next few days they monitored her very closely. She still wasn't having very much urine output so they decided to try a different medication and increased her blood pressure medications to see if more blood flow to her kidneys would help her urinate. Labs had shown that the inflammation levels from her NEC were going down and she was responding nicely to the antibiotics.

Later that day she had the wettest diaper she had ever had. I never thought I would say "YAY for Pee!" but it was such a relief that she had finally urinated. It seemed like she was starting to improve and her NEC was clearing up. They did have to increase her sedation medications because she kept trying to fight her ventilator and breathe over it. Most people; like I did, would think that would be a good thing but they needed all of her energy going towards "resting and growing" and not trying to breathe on her own right now. They tried switching her to a different type of ventilator to see if that would help but her oxygen needs got worse so they switched her back to the jet ventilator. After tweaking the settings on her ventilator a little bit, and after the sedation medications kicked in, she relaxed and stopped fighting.

September 29th, 2017

Day of life- 19 Gestational age-26.1 weeks

Today our community has organized a fundraiser called "Laps for Loretta." My husband's mom works for the school district and is a cross country coach. While we were all at the hospital, the cross country team decided they wanted to organize a run for Loretta to raise awareness and money to help with medical costs. This run was taking place tonight. My husband and I did not attend as it was two hours from the hospital and we didn't want to leave Loretta's side but my husband's mom said the turnout was amazing. There was so much love and support for our family that it warmed our hearts knowing how many people cared and were praying just as hard as we were for our little girl.

Over the next week Loretta's oxygen needs started increasing and she became very restless. They tried to get a spinal tap to check to see if she could possibly have meningitis but they were unable to collect any cervical fluid. They did a supra pubic tap to see if she had an infection and started antibiotics while we waited for the results. We were terrified as we awaited the results and they came back that Loretta had pneumonia. I was devastated. It seemed like just one thing after another kept hitting her. How could such a tiny human being fight pneumonia with very sick, under-developed lungs? We were so worried for her as the doctors told us that all we could at this point was give her antibiotics and let her rest. She was already on a diuretic to help her pee off any fluid that may be on her lungs and she still had the pain & sedation meds on board.

I tried to distract myself a little by decorating her room for Halloween. I decided I was going to try to scare the pneumonia right out of her. I think she had the most festive room in the Unit because all of the nurses kept coming in to look. I decided if my baby can't be home for the holidays then I was going to make her room her home and make the best of it. It was also a little more comforting to me also as I spent most of my time in her room and was tired of looking at blank walls. We needed to make the best of the situation and being we knew we would be here for at least a few more months; we made it our home.

After being on antibiotics for a week for her pneumonia; Loretta's oxygen needs hadn't improved very much so they started her on surfactant and dexamethasone. The surfactant was a medication to help lubricate her lungs in case her air sacs were tight from being on the ventilator and the dexamethasone was a steroid that was supposed to help open up those air sacs. Later that evening her oxygen saturations started improving.

October 10th, 2017

Day of Life- 30   Gestational Age: 27.5 weeks

Loretta hit two pounds for her weight!! She likes to kangaroo with mommy and daddy, kicking her legs, flinging her eye cloth off of her eyes, blowing spit bubbles, stretching, putting her hands above her head, gripping our fingers, grabbing onto her breathing tube, sleeping and holding her breath which makes all of her alarms go off. She is the strongest little girl I know and I truly believe she is a miracle. I can't believe how far she has come and how much she has overcome. She has been through so much but is doing well. I get emotional thinking of everything she has endured so far and how she just keeps kicking butt. She is a true warrior and if she can fight all of this and be so strong; then so could we.

A couple of days later, they took her broviac line out. She finished the steroid for her lungs and her oxygen saturations continued to improve. Her doctor decided that he felt it was time to try taking her breathing tube out and see if she could breathe on her own with just a CPAP mask. Her ventilator was showing that she was taking a lot of breaths on her own and she had outgrown her breathing tube so it had an air leak. She was also constantly tugging on her breathing tube anyways so now seemed like a good time to try.

Loretta did great switching over to the CPAP and her oxygen needs went down. Her saturations were very good and the doctors were impressed. We were so proud of her and it was such an amazing feeling to be able to hold her with only a CPAP mask on and not having to worry about her breathing tube coming out.

The next day, Loretta even started to suck on a pacifier; she was able to do so now that she didn't have the breathing tube in. She was now on day five of being off of her breathing tube and her oxygen needs were starting to go back up. Her lungs were getting tired of breathing on their own, even with another dose of steroids on board.

I was sitting there thinking of how proud I was that she was able to even make it five days on CPAP and that it was okay if she needed to rest and grow longer so her lungs could develop more. I was so proud of her and could tell she wanted to do it on her own.

Suddenly, I heard her alarms start going off and nurses and doctors came rushing into her room. I stood back in panic watching as they surrounded her. They took her CPAP mask off and started giving her manual breaths of air. My worst fear came true; she stopped breathing.

What felt like an eternity was only a couple of minutes and she started breathing on her own again. One of the nurses noticed me falling apart and asked if I would wait outside. They put a breathing tube back in and put her back on the ventilator. Once Loretta was stable again, her doctor came out and explained that she had a few episodes where she had stopped breathing and it was more than likely because she wasn't ready to breathe on her own yet. She did very well being off of the breathing tube for the past five days but her lungs got tired and she just needed more time to develop, so in the meantime she would be on the ventilator.

I thanked her doctors and nurses for being there as fast as they were and saving my little girl. There aren't enough words I could use to explain how grateful I am of her care team. Not only do they give her the BEST care, but they also care about us as parents also. Without me realizing it they had called the social worker to come in and speak to me. The nurses could tell that her episode took a toll on me and wanted to make sure I had all the resources that I needed. When the social worker walked in, I hung up the phone with my husband and broke down as I talked to her. I felt every emotion pouring out of me, exactly like the day we lost our son. I was so afraid I was going to lose her too.

Teddy

The day Teddy died was one of the hardest days of my life. I like to think I'm a strong person; I have been through a lot in my life, but this might just break me. It feels like a heavy weight is on my chest. It's hard to breathe at times and this pain I have, I haven't experienced before. I feel like my brain is scattered everywhere. I can't focus and often lose my train of thought. I sit and stare zoned out, feeling numb. I grieve for my son. I miss him and I hurt because of the fact that my daughter will have to grow up without her twin. I often wonder if she'll still feel that connection with him when she gets older. Will she remember him?

At first I told myself that we wouldn't tell her about Teddy until she was a lot older unless she did have some kind of connection and brought it up to us sooner, but then my husband and I decided it is important that we cherish Teddy's memory. He was our baby, he was alive and he was here. He fought like a true warrior and as painful as this whole situation is, we can't just ignore it. We need to talk about it and it is important for Loretta to know she has a twin.

One of Loretta's primary nurses in the NICU, that also was the nurse assigned to Teddy, bought Loretta a teddy bear that had Teddy's name engraved on it with their birthday. This was one of the most thoughtful gifts anyone has ever given us. This was something Loretta could hold onto & snuggle with when she gets older to hopefully comfort her. So we made it a ritual that when we celebrate Loretta's milestones or holidays we would include Teddy into the pictures. This is our way of cherishing his memory and bringing a little comfort to our broken hearts.

We had Teddy cremated and kept his remains in my daughter's NICU room so that he would be close to her. Being that we were practically living at the hospital, we wanted him there with us. Teddy's nurses had put together a memorial box for us which contained his blanket, wristbands, teddy bear, hand & footprints, pictures and a lock of his hair. This box is so special to us; it's all we have left of our little boy. One day, I am hoping we will share this with Loretta once she is much older.

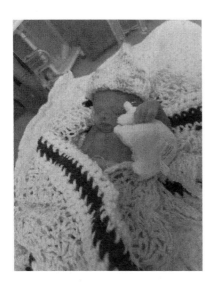

A letter for Teddy,

As I sit here and stare at our beautiful daughter's face, I wonder what it would be like if you were here. She looks just like you. My heart aches as it's a constant reminder. Every day is a constant reminder; from walking into those same doors and down the same halls past your old room. It brings back all of the pain, fear and uncertainty all over again. Did we make the right decision? Was it the best decision? Would you have gotten better and proved them wrong like she has?

I don't think I've ever hurt this badly. I've loved you from the moment I found out we we're blessed with you. I fell even more in love with every ultrasound picture, every kick and every butterfly in my stomach.

Holding you for the very first and last time that I would be able to was so emotional and confusing. Why was this happening to us? Should I have done things differently? Could I have fought harder? These are the guilts I live with every day.

Deep down I know I gave it my all, I fought hard and would have continued to do so as long as I possibly could. But I couldn't, my body failed me. It was no longer possible. Even though I still had the will, determination and fight left in me; my body didn't. My body failed you. I am so sorry baby that you went through this. I am so sorry I failed you. You should be here.

I wonder what her life will be like without you. I wonder if she has that connection already being that you were her twin. Only time will tell, and I pray one day I'll know what to say and how to explain. She's been through so much and she's a fighter, just like you were. She's fighting for the both of you Teddy.

It's heart wrenching when people ask "how many children do you have?" Not knowing a simple question like that devastates us every single time. The truth is that we have one baby here and one angel baby ahead of us.

The Power of Prayer

After pulling myself together after talking to the social worker, I just prayed. I prayed the lord would help Loretta get better. I prayed that he was watching over Teddy. I prayed that he would give me the strength to get through this roller coaster ride. I needed to be strong for our little girl. I know others were praying too. Our church, community, family, friends, coworkers, staff at the hospital and people we didn't even know prayed for us. I found strength in the power of their prayers. I felt like at that moment we were living our lives on a prayer. All of our hope and worries were in God's hands. I knew he had a bigger plan than I could understand at that moment but I had faith he would keep his healing hands on Loretta.

After letting Loretta rest for a couple days, Loretta's blood gas lab work came back and her CO2 levels were really high. Her right lung had collapsed. Her kidney function labs also weren't good and she had stopped urinating again. Once again we were punched in the gut. The doctors ordered to give her Lasix again to help her urinate and they took blood work and collected a sample from her breathing tube and sent for a culture. They started antibiotics and another steroid to hopefully help her kidney function; also stopping her feedings. They had to put an IV & PICC line in and also placed a catheter again. Six hours later they took another X-ray to check her lungs and it had shown that her left lung had now collapsed. Her hemoglobin was also down so they gave her another blood transfusion. My poor baby was being poked and prodded all day long and dealing with collapsed lungs. My heart ached as there was nothing I could do to help her except pray. The respiratory therapist came in and adjusted her ventilator settings to give her longer breaths and after her blood transfusion was done she finally started to improve.

The next morning she had another echocardiogram and head ultrasound to check her heart and brain. The doctor stated they both looked good which was the best news I had heard in a while. I felt that the last several days were just one bad thing after another so I was very happy to hear this. Her head ultrasound showed that the old blood that was on her brain was starting to resolve or disappear. There was a small amount of swelling but they believed it was from the blood resolving so they weren't worried about it. The CRP lab they drew to check inflammation in her body was high so they stated they were going to monitor that closely for infection.

The next couple of weeks were a rollercoaster of ups and downs with her oxygen needs. She had a set back where she was back to 100% oxygen needs; meaning she wasn't breathing on her own at all. That night while I was holding her, my mama instincts kicked in that something just wasn't right. I had a gut feeling that she had pneumonia again so I asked the doctors to order another culture from her breathing tube. I knew they had just done

one last week and it was okay but something was just telling me they needed to do it again; so her doctor respected my wishes and did the test. They also started antibiotics while we waited for the lab culture. When the results came back it confirmed she did have pneumonia again. My poor baby wasn't even two months old yet and already had pneumonia 3 times and collapsed lungs on both sides.

November 7th, 2017

Day of life: 58   Gestational Age: 31.5 weeks

     Loretta weighed in at 3lbs 8oz this morning.
Normally we would be ecstatic that she gained weight but
she had gained too much weight overnight. She had
gained 10 ounces overnight and was very puffy looking.
She was still at 100% on her oxygen needs and not
urinating. After another round of Lasix and Bumex she
started urinating later that evening. Her blood results
came back from that morning and she tested positive for
CMV. CMV is a virus that is very common and can
infect anyone. Once CMV is in a person's body, it stays
there for life and can reactivate from time to time; kind of
like a cold sore for example. For a baby like Loretta with
a very weak immune system; CMV could be deadly. Her
doctors stated that she had acquired it after she was
born which was better than if she would have acquired it
in utero and had been born with it. A baby born with
CMV could potentially lead to deafness, blindness,
intellectual disability, small head size, lack of
coordination, seizures and weakness in muscles.

The next morning they placed a PICC line in and started her on Ganciclovir for the CMV. This antibiotic was very rigorous and is often used on chemo patients. I think I about collapsed when they told me this. I was very hesitant about them giving her a chemo drug but her doctor reassured me it was on the "less potent" end of the chemo drugs and that she would need to be on this medication for 30 days to help treat her CMV.

How could such a little baby that only weighed about three pounds survive a chemo drug? And she was still on the other antibiotics for her pneumonia. I was so frightened but gave them consent to do it. Once again, I prayed to God that I was making the right decision and that he would keep his healing hands on her.

At this point Loretta was the oldest baby in the "Small Baby Neighborhood" in the NICU. It was time to move her out to the "General Population" unit of the NICU but her nurses wanted to give it a few more days so they could monitor her extra close being she just started the antibiotic for CMV and she was also getting another blood, platelet and red blood cell transfusion.

The next day Loretta, graduated from the Small Baby Neighborhood and moved to the General Population; literally from one end of the unit to the other. Room #45 to Room#1. It was a little bit of an adjustment for us because we went from a unit that was very quiet and dark to a unit that was busier, nosier and brighter. Instead of having one nurse to ourselves we had to share a nurse with another baby next door. Being on the new side did have its perks though. For the first time she would be able to sleep with her incubator top popped completely open. I cannot explain the fullness my heart felt that I could now go over and bend over to kiss her. I couldn't do this before with the incubator closed. We could only put our hand in the small hole to touch her unless we got her out to hold her. The nurse stated if she did well maintaining her body temperature on her own that they would move her to a crib after a couple of days. I couldn't believe that my baby would actually be going to a crib. She seemed like such a big girl and was making such good progress.

Loretta was outgrowing her breathing tube again so it had a huge air leak and the respiratory therapist had to keep adjusting the ventilator settings to compensate for the leak. Her doctor decided that when she was done with her CMV medication that we would try to take her breathing tube out again and put her on CPAP. I was excited but mainly terrified. It was good we were making progress but I was terrified we would go through what we went through last time when she stopped breathing. It had been weighing on my mind all day so later that evening our nurse asked if my husband and I wanted to give Loretta a sponge bath. "Of course!" we exclaimed. After 66 days in the NICU we were able to give our baby girl a bed bath for the first time and we also weighed her in at 3lbs 15 ½ ounces. We had almost made it to four pounds! We couldn't believe how big our baby girl was and all of the new things we were able to do with her.

Later that evening the doctor came in and stated that despite the fact she was still on the medication for her CMV, they have decided to try switching her to CPAP tomorrow after a dose of steroids. They felt that she was ready and they weren't able to make any more adjustments on her ventilator to compensate for the air leak. He reassured me that they would be all set up and ready to go so if she wasn't able to breathe on her own they would be prepared to put in a larger breathing tube.

The next day came and they tried pulling her tube out. She did breathe on her own for a while but she was working really hard so they decided to put the bigger breathing tube in and try again after a couple weeks. She needed more time to grow and develop. With the new breathing tube going in, she had more secretions in her tube so they tested it and the culture came back that she had gotten pneumonia again. They decided they would treat her with steroid nebulizers this time which helped tremendously. One thing after another but our brave little girl is a true fighter; a warrior princess.

Home for the Holidays?

Loretta hit four pounds right before Thanksgiving Day. We spend Thanksgiving with our family in Loretta's NICU room. She is becoming more alert and active now that she isn't on as much morphine and ativan to sedate her. Thanks to the Ronald McDonald house and volunteers, we were able to have a Thanksgiving Dinner there.

We had met another family that had recently had a 24 weeker that was in the NICU. The parents had shown me a picture of her and I immediately broke down into tears. I had flashbacks to when Loretta was that small and I hadn't realized how much this whole situation has impacted me. I've been so focused on Loretta that I didn't realize I was also struggling with PTSD. I gave the parents a hug and told them I was there if they needed anything. I completely understood and wanted to be there for them. I couldn't believe it had already been 2 ½ months since we had been in the NICU. I had shown them a picture of Loretta and told them a little of her story hoping it would give them hope that things do get better.

The next day I couldn't help but think about the family that we had met. I wanted to be able to do more for parents that were going through exactly what we were going through. I ran into them later that day when I went to get lunch and we exchanged phone numbers. We started talking more and became friends. I could tell they appreciated the advice and feedback from what we had went through. I wanted to help them in any way I could and most importantly wanted to make sure they didn't lose hope.

When I returned to Loretta's room the nurse had stated that she had a yeast infection on her breathing tube so they were going to start her on another antibiotic to treat that. She stated that Loretta more than likely got the yeast infection because of all of the other antibiotics she had been on. The ophthalmologist also had come by to do Loretta's eye exam and stated that they needed to monitor her closely because she had developed Retinopathy which was common in premature babies in which the retina could potentially detach from the eye if the condition got worse. At this point they would monitor with weekly checks and only do treatment if it progressed.

A couple of days went by and Loretta began tugging on her breathing tube again. Now that she wasn't as sedated, she was more aware that she had a tube going down her throat. She was now shoving her hands in her mouth around her breathing tube and her doctor felt that it was time to try taking her tube out again. They gave her steroids again and removed her tube. They put the CPAP mask on her and she took off! She was doing it on her own. She was breathing on her own! I was so excited for her but wanted to be realistic to not get discouraged if her lungs got tired again and she had to go back on the breathing tube.

After a few days, she was still doing very well on the CPAP machine and her pulmonologist was very happy with how her lungs sounded. Loretta had become very agitated which was a side effect from being on the steroids so I spent most of the day holding her as that was the only thing that would comfort her. The steroids were a huge help for her lungs but it wasn't easy watching the side effects.

December 7th, 2017

Day of life-88   Gestational Age-36 weeks

      Since Loretta has been on CPAP for a week and is doing well, they have decided to switch her to high flow oxygen. This means she gets rid of her CPAP mask and will now just have a nose cannula. She tolerated the switch very well and I think she enjoyed having the CPAP mask off of her face. She still tries to pull the nose cannula off but it is a lot better than the mask. She is now completely off all of her antibiotics and steroids and also tried the bottle for the first time today! She was only able to get a few drops but she did it. This was huge progress for her.

They tried the bottle again a week later and she was able to take about 7 milliliters; which is equivalent to about a teaspoon. The speech therapist came to work with Loretta on eating and suggested we do a swallow study to make sure she wasn't aspirating the milk into her lungs.

The next day we did the swallow study and it showed that she was indeed aspirating both thin and thick liquids into her lungs so we were advised to stop bottling her and give it time. She was still getting all of her feedings through her feeding tube and just needed more time to develop and learn how to suck and swallow correctly.

With Christmas approaching, I began to take down the Thanksgiving decorations and put up Christmas decorations instead. One of the nurses came by and said that she had spotted Santa in the NICU so I hurried up and put a pretty dress on Loretta just in time as Santa walked into her room. We were able to get a picture with him and he even left her a present! It was so nice that they did this for families in the NICU; I felt like it put a little "normal" back into our lives.

On Christmas day our family came and spent Christmas in the NICU with Loretta. We opened her presents from Santa and decided we would wait on our gifts until she came home and then we would celebrate at that time. We were so thankful this year that we were blessed with our Christmas Miracle. It seemed that the rollercoaster may have started to slow down and that she was finally starting to improve.

A New Year

January 4th, 2018

Day of life: 116   Gestational Age: 40 weeks

Today is our baby girl's due date! I am filled with all kinds of emotions today. I am thankful and blessed that Loretta has come this far. She has gone through so much and has overcome it all. I know she has a long road ahead of her but we choose to focus on what's happening now and she's doing amazing considering the circumstances. I am also grieving today. I am missing Teddy and wishing he was still here. I feel robbed that I didn't get to finish my pregnancy. The guilt sets in that I couldn't carry my babies to full term. The reality was that I only made it just over half way through my pregnancy. I literally went through hell and back fighting for my babies and delivered two micro-preemies. I have learned so much about strength and courage from my babies and my faith has only gotten stronger. I felt selfish because of the fact that I was angry with God before for taking my son. I just wanted him back but now was feeling selfish thinking I should be grateful that I still have my daughter. I now know that it was not selfishness; I am simply grieving. While trying to process things today, I wrote a letter for my daughter:

My princess warrior,

Today is the day. Today is your due date. Today, you are also 116 days old. You are the strongest, most beautiful little girl in the world. You are so brave and have overcome so much. You've already dealt with more than most do in a lifetime and you don't even know it yet; but we do. We all do. You are loved so much by so many.

You are my hero, my strength and my pride. You started with every odd stacked against you and have overcome what we were told would be impossible. You have left doctors baffled and scratching their heads. You are proof that miracles DO happen and my faith is so much stronger because of you.

It is not fair that you were born 17 weeks early and had a rough start, but this does not define you. This is your story. A story about a warrior princess that can overcome anything because she has already had to. You are strong and brave. You bring so much happiness to our lives. We love you, always and forever, to the moon and back!

The next couple of weeks we focused on Loretta growing and gaining weight. She had hit 7lbs, was stable on her oxygen, her brain bleeds had completely resolved on their own without surgery, the retinopathy in her eyes looked like it had improved a little and she passed her hearing test. We still were unable to work on bottling because she was still aspirating it into her lungs. Speech therapy recommended that a genetic doctor see Loretta as they felt that there may be an underlying condition based on facial features and the fact she was having so much trouble swallowing. I felt kind of offended at first as I felt that they were saying something was wrong with my baby and she is perfect in my eyes, but after I realized I was being emotional and that it couldn't hurt I agreed with them.

The Genetics team came in and requested to draw lab work on Loretta. I gave consent and they stated it would take a couple days for the results to come back. In the meantime her doctor recommended that we have a g-tube placed. This whole time her feeding tube has been either down her nose or through her mouth and if we did the g-tube procedure it would go directly into her belly from her abdomen. This would mean that she could go home faster and work on eating from home. We were skeptical about putting her under anesthesia and doing another procedure but after talking it over for a few days and learning how the g-tube would work; we agreed to the surgery. We just wanted to finally be able to bring our baby girl home.

The results from the genetic testing came back and the genetic doctor and counselor came to Loretta's room to talk with me. They explained that Loretta has a deletion of chromosome 7q11.22; which is also a part of the AUTS2 gene. As of right now they are unsure of what that will mean for her as there isn't much for research on it yet. It could potentially lead to developmental delays, high or low muscle tone, blindness, deafness, dwarfism, speech impairments or feeding difficulties; but those were things we wouldn't know until later on. We were devastated to hear this news. Our baby has already been through so much and I felt like I was being told that she would never be able to do these things. I cried for several days praying that this won't affect her. For now, we don't know; but what I do know is she is perfect. She is a fighter and has already proved she can overcome things that doctors thought she wouldn't. I have faith and I believe in her that she can overcome this too. We will do whatever it takes to help her and get her the help she needs. This doesn't define who she is or what she can do. She is stronger than this and I have to be strong for her. We are fighters and we don't give up.

I realized that I have had these types of mindsets throughout our whole journey through the NICU. No matter how much we felt like we were being beaten down; we chose to rise above and I honestly believe our faith had a huge part in that. We have had many people tell us how proud they are of us for how we handled our situation; but any good parent would do the same. When you have babies your whole world changes and you will go through hell and back to protect them and give them whatever they need; especially when you are a NICU parent.

January 16th, 2018

Day of life: 128   Gestational Age: 41.5 Weeks

        Today is Loretta's G-Tube procedure. I have
mixed emotions. Part of me feels awful that we are putting
her through a procedure and that she will have to have a
feeding tube into her stomach but this will allow her to go
home in a couple of weeks. Hopefully she will only need
the feeding tube for a few months. It's scary to watch as
they poke her for labs, put IVs back in and re-intubate
her. This takes me back to before when this was a daily
routine and we were constantly living in fear if she'd
survive; but she's such a fighter and as worried as I was,
there was still a sense that everything would be okay. I
walked with the nurse as she rolled Loretta's crib to
surgery. As they prepped her the surgeon explained to
me exactly what would be taking place. I felt a little more
at ease and completely trusted them with my daughter. I
can't say enough good things about the staff at
Children's hospital. The professionalism and kindness

behind each one of them is inspiring. Loretta's nurse came out and hugged me and told me everything would be okay and she would be back in a while to check on me.

Loretta's surgery only took about 30 minutes and the surgeon came out and said everything went good and Loretta did great. I cried tears of happiness. My baby girl continues to amaze me with her strength each and every day. I walked back down to Loretta's room and waited for them to bring her back. As soon as she came back, I just wanted to snuggle her up but was encouraged to wait until the next day so she could rest. She was uncomfortable and her surgery site was tender so it was best not to move her around.

The next morning, Loretta was feeling much better from her procedure and during the roundings meeting her doctor actual mentioned the word "discharge." My face lit up with excitement as I knew we were finally getting close. The doctors stated that they were shooting to discharge her the following week and there would be many classes that my husband and I would need to take before she came home so they would start getting those set up.

Over the next several days, my husband and I took many classes. We learned how to use her g-tube, feeding pump and bags, syringes to administer her medications through her g-tube and how to use a danny sling which is what she would need to sleep in because of her reflux. They explained how to use the sling and that her bed would need to be slanted at an angle while she slept. We got acquainted with her oxygen tank and how that would work at home along with the monitors that would go along with it. We also took infant CPR and started packing up her NICU room. I couldn't believe the day we would take her home was almost here. My husband and I went home that night to do last minute things around the house and prepare for her coming home. We couldn't believe the next time we would be home it would be with our daughter.

A few days later, Loretta passed her car seat test and just needed to pass her sleep study before she would be able to go home. We were very anxious as that was the last thing from keeping her from coming home and we prayed she would pass. The next morning they collected her sleep study machine and we anxiously waited for the results. My husband and I went to lunch and when we came back our nurse told us SHE PASSED!! Loretta was ready to go home and would be discharged the next morning. My husband and I were emotional as we thought about this whole journey. We had been in the NICU for 4 ½ months on top of the 10 days that I was hospitalized prior to delivery. It had been one crazy ride but we had made it and were ready for a new beginning.

A New Beginning

My husband and I woke up this morning filled with all types of emotions. Today is discharge day! Our baby girl has been in the NICU for 136 days with many ups and downs. We have witnessed and been through things no parent should have to go through. We are overwhelmed with emotions from tears of joy to tears of sadness knowing we have to say goodbye. We were so happy to start a new beginning at home with our daughter, but also sad to be saying goodbye to all of the NICU staff that has become our family. For 136 days these people have cared for our little girl, befriended us, picked us up when we were down, held our hand as we cried and made things as easy on us as they possibly could. Without them, today would not be possible. Today is the day that Loretta will go outside, take a car ride, see the world outside of the NICU and finally go home for the very first time. So many of the NICU staff took time out of their days to come wish us well and say goodbye. Our little miracle had touched so many hearts and we could tell they were filled with emotions too.

One of our primary nurses came in to work that day because she knew Loretta was being discharged. A couple of months ago she said that her wish for her birthday this year was that Loretta would get to go home and ironically today was her birthday; the same day we were being discharged. She walked Loretta and I out to the front door as we waited for my husband to pull the truck around. We were both quiet and couldn't believe this day was finally here. When the truck pulled up she helped me bring Loretta outside and get her all buckled in. Before we left we shed some tears and gave her big hugs. We couldn't have gotten through this journey without our primary nurses and I am honestly terrified to go home without them but they reassured us that we would do great.

After we said our goodbyes, I climbed into the backseat and sat next to our baby girl and my husband pulled away. We were terrified. Were we ready for this? I carefully watched her oxygen saturations on her monitor as we headed home. It felt weird to be going "home" when the hospital had been our home for the last 4 ½ months; we had forgot what it felt like to be at our home. When we arrived at home; we took our baby girl into the living room and sat there for a little while in disbelief. We couldn't believe we were actually home. We couldn't believe everything that had happened.

We requested no visitors at all the first week we were home so we could finally have quality alone time with our daughter. This was the first time we had been alone with her and we wanted to get a routine down and have time to process things. After a week we started letting immediate family members come over as long as they weren't sick or had been exposed to anyone that was sick. Anyone who entered our home had to stop and wash their hands before going near Loretta. We were on lock down per doctor's orders as it was crucial she didn't get sick. If Loretta got even a common cold, it could potentially put her right back in the hospital. The last thing we wanted was her sick and back in the hospital so we didn't take her anywhere except her follow up doctor appointments.

The first month being home was chaotic and stressful. We had white boards on the wall to keep track of her feeding and medication times so both my husband and I were on the same page. Every two hours was filled with something that needed to be done. After a couple of weeks we had gotten the hang of it and it became easier. My husband had to return to work and my mother-in-law took a month off of work to help me. We stayed busy with many follow up appointments with Loretta's specialists. She was doing well & thriving at home.

It has now been four months since we have been home and Loretta is doing very well. She has come off of her oxygen during the day and now only wears it at night. She sees occupational and physical therapy weekly, works with the feeding clinic, has a dietician follow her closely to make sure she is getting all her nutrients and is gaining weight properly and she is thriving. She is a very strong willed & stubborn little girl; some would say like her mom. I am so proud of her and am so blessed to be her mommy. Our journey is not over and we have a long road ahead of us, but when you have faith; nothing is worth giving up on. We will continue to take it day by day and focus on what today brings, because after all, we are just living on a prayer.

Insights

As a NICU mom, it has changed my perspective on a lot of things. It has made me a stronger person but has also made me a more sensitive person. I remember I would cringe when a nurse would tell me to "take a break" or "enjoy your sleep now because once you go home, you won't get any." To them, these were words of advice. They truly did care and wanted us as parents to take care of ourselves too; but when you are a NICU parent, you look forward to those sleepless nights at home. And the truth is that if you are not in the hospital room with your baby during the middle of the night; you are lying awake in your bed restless, worrying about if your baby will make it through the night or not. You are afraid to leave and take a break because of how fast things change in the NICU. One minute your baby could be stable and the next could be the scariest moment of your life.

During our stay in the NICU, we were fortunate enough to be able to stay in The Ronald McDonald house; which was one floor above the NICU. We lived two hours from the hospital and if it wasn't for the Ronald McDonald house, we would have been traveling back and forth every day. I had many sleepless nights and was fortunate enough to be able to walk downstairs and go into my daughter's room to check on her. I knew she was in the best care possible; but it still put my mind to ease to check. I had a hard time leaving her room so I rarely did. I was so afraid something bad would happen so I was there all day, every day. The nurses would have to remind me to go get lunch and tried to encourage me to go outside for a walk. I was completely consumed with what was happening to my daughter that nothing else mattered. My priority was to get her through this.

My advice for NICU parents would be to sign up for primary nurses. This means that your baby will have a better chance of being assigned to that nurse if they are working. We had four primary nurses for our daughter and it made it a lot easier on us. We got familiar with how our nurses did things and we felt more comfortable asking questions and getting involved. By the end of our 136 day NICU stay, our primary nurses had become our family. We were so close to them and couldn't have gotten through our journey without them. Well, we couldn't have gotten through our NICU journey without any of the NICU nurses or providers that cared for our daughter. We loved them all, but our primaries couldn't be replaced. They had picked us up when we were at our lowest, held us while we cried, encouraged us, taught us how to be involved with cares and became our friends. Two of our primary nurses were working the night our son passed away. We couldn't have gotten through that night without them. The impact that they had on us had brought us to tears while we were being discharged. We would miss them.

I would also tell you to speak up when you have a gut instinct on something. It took me awhile to become comfortable enough to speak up to doctors if I thought something wasn't right; after all, what did I know? But it was so important! I distinctly remember the first mama instinct I had. It was a few weeks after we had been in the NICU and I felt that something with my daughter was "off." This wasn't easy to detect because she couldn't cry with her breathing tube in but something just told me that something was wrong. I had noticed throughout that day that she had more secretions in her breathing tube and the nurses had to suction her more often. I had approached the care team with my concerns so they ran a culture of my daughter's breathing tube and a couple of days later it came back that she had pneumonia; before she was even showing signs. Our mama instincts are powerful and we know things before they are apparent, so don't be afraid to speak up! This helped my baby tremendously as she was treated before her symptoms had even started. We know our babies better than anyone else.

I struggled at first feeling like the nurses were more of a mama than I was because there wasn't much that I could do at that time other than hold her; but this was so important. My baby needed to feel me; feel my heart beat and feel my skin. This was something the nurses weren't able to do, but I could. So as intimidating as the situation is, hold your baby if you can. They need you and I promise you that they know that it is you. I also suggest talking with other NICU parents. They understand what you are going through more than anyone else and it can be comforting for both you and them. There are also social workers, chaplains and many other support contacts the nurses can get for you if you need someone to talk to. So remember: speak up, get in daily snuggles if you can, get involved with cares and take care of yourself too!

My advice for friends or family members of NICU parents would be to be patient with us. The NICU is traumatizing and it changes us. We will probably never be the same again. We may stop the daily texts because we are so consumed with what is going on in the NICU; but we so much appreciate those phone calls or text messages from you that let us know you care. We barely have the energy to pull ourselves into bed at night so please be understanding if you don't hear much from us during this difficult time. Please don't get discouraged if you can't meet our babies right away. Most NICU's have strict rules on visitors and only allow so many per day, depending on the condition of the baby. It is critical that our babies don't get sick as most of them have very sick, underdeveloped lungs and no immune system. Depending on the prematurity of the baby, they are easily overstimulated so can't have loud noises or lights on.

A question I was asked from family and friends frequently while in the NICU was "is there anything I can do for you?" At the time I was too afraid to ask or burden anyone, or maybe I just didn't know, but yes, food is great! I had several times when people would drop off a meal and I appreciated it so much because I often forgot to go and get something to eat and to be honest the cafeteria food gets old after a while. I also remember my mother in-law going to my house and cleaning it before we came home from the NICU because I didn't want to leave my daughter but I was paranoid of "germs" and the four and a half months worth of dust in my house because I hadn't been home to clean it. Coming home to a clean house was a huge weight off my shoulders. Even a simple text message to let us know you are thinking of us can take our mind off of the NICU, even if it's only for a second, it means a lot. These were all huge things that meant so much to me.

Please use words of encouragement when talking to us about our babies. For example; "Your baby looks great and I can tell she is growing!" Reminding us that our babies are super small is kind of like picking the scab back open. We aren't naive; we know they are small but sometimes it's painful to keep hearing it. We appreciate hearing how well they are doing or how good they look. I know I also appreciated when people would comment that our baby looked like me or my husband. Because she was born so prematurely, it took a long time for her features to stand out or for her to grow out of the "prematurity" look. I know this might seem silly, but trust me; I became a sensitive mama bear that was ready to attack anyone that was going to make me feel like something was wrong with my baby. I'm sure other mamas feel the same way and want to hear nothing but positive comments.

I know I personally appreciated when others would acknowledge my baby boy that had passed away. As painful as it is, I find comfort in others talking to me about it and acknowledging that he was my baby boy and that he was here. I know it's not always a comfortable subject to bring up but speaking for myself, it helped me grieve and did more good than anything.

When we get home from the NICU; please give us time to re-adjust to our new life. When I got home, all I wanted to do was snuggle my baby. I wanted to be the one to change her dirty diapers, comfort her when she cried, get the most snuggles and build that one on one bond. In the NICU, I did participate in cares and changing her diapers but there was usually always a nurse there to help. When I got home, I wanted to do it ALL and ALL on my own. That is what helped me feel more like I was her mom. Also, please don't question our parenting or why we are being overbearing. I remember being told by a family member that our baby needed to be exposed a little so she could build her immune system. My mama bear almost came roaring out as the thoughts crossed my mind that a simple cold could potentially hospitalize my baby again and that she would have plenty of time to be "exposed" once she got older and healthier. We also had a lot of people that wanted to come and visit once we got home. We appreciated that people wanted to see us and meet our baby but please don't get offended if we say no. In our case, we were under strict doctor's orders and were pretty much on house arrest. Our baby came home on oxygen and a feeding tube and it was still very crucial that she didn't get sick; so we still kind of lived like we did in the NICU. Except we didn't have all of the doctors and nurses there to help us and we were scared shitless. My point is, our babies just had the fight of their life, literally. We will be overprotective, overbearing and crazy at times but we have every right to be. We are only doing what we believe is in the best interest for our baby; just like any other parent would do. The most important thing to remember is that we need you. We need your support and to know that we aren't alone. So please be patient and understanding while we get through this crazy ride.

I do want to give a huge shout-out and thank you from the bottom of my heart to Children's Hospital and the entire NICU care team for saving our daughter and helping us get through the roller coaster ride. We couldn't have done it without you and there are no words to express how thankful we are for each and every one of you! I also want to thank The Ronald McDonald House for giving us one of the best gifts we could have been given during a situation like this; which was a home away from home. We thank our families, friends and communities for all of their love, support and prayers. We love you all and are so grateful! If you are interested in donating to help families in situations like mine, there are many non-profit organizations including The Potato Head Project, The Ronald McDonald House, March of Dimes, and so many others. These were just a few of the ones that helped us through our NICU journey and we are so grateful!

I'm hoping that my insights are helpful. It's not easy to understand the NICU life unless you have lived through it and hopefully this will give just a little bit of insight to what parents go through or why they feel strongly about certain things that maybe others disagree on. Just don't argue with us. I'm kidding. I'm hoping I haven't offended anyone and you were able to find a little humor in some of my insights. Parents in the NICU; don't give up hope. No matter how dark things get, there is a light at the end of the tunnel. Our little humans are so much stronger than they may seem. Sending love to you all!

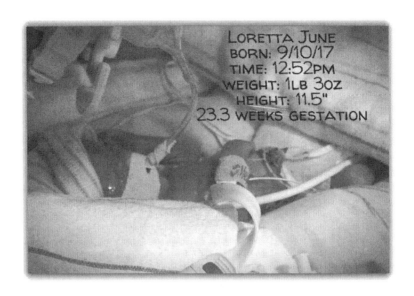

LORETTA JUNE
BORN: 9/10/17
TIME: 12:52PM
WEIGHT: 1LB 3OZ
HEIGHT: 11.5"
23.3 WEEKS GESTATION

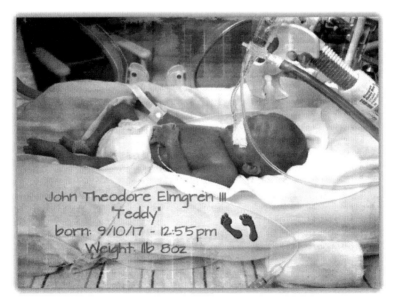

John Theodore Elmgren III
"Teddy"
born: 9/10/17 - 12:55pm
Weight: 1lb 8oz

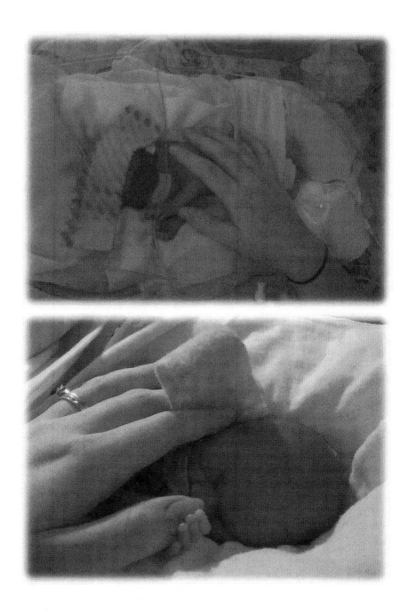

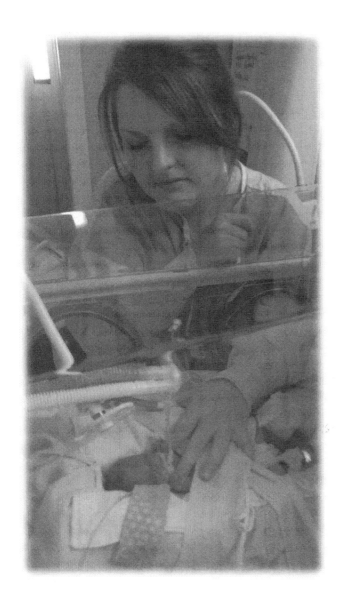

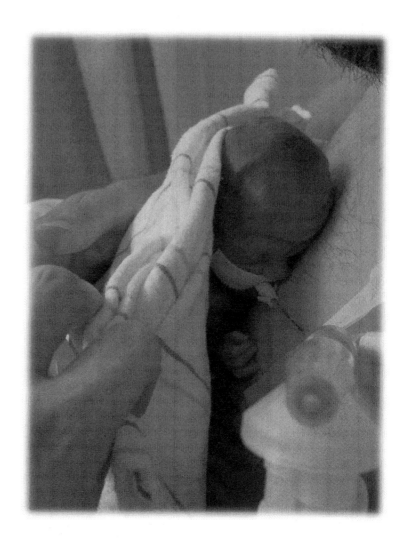

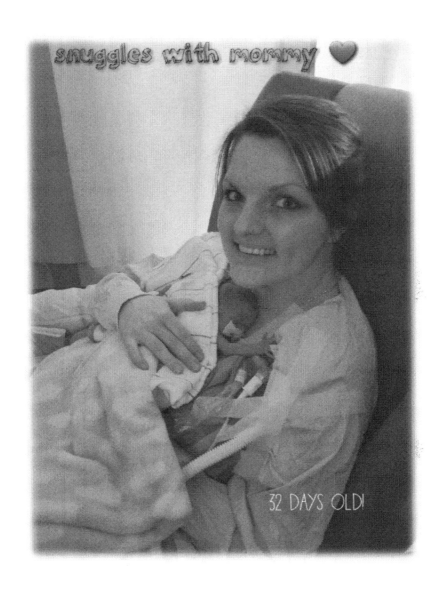

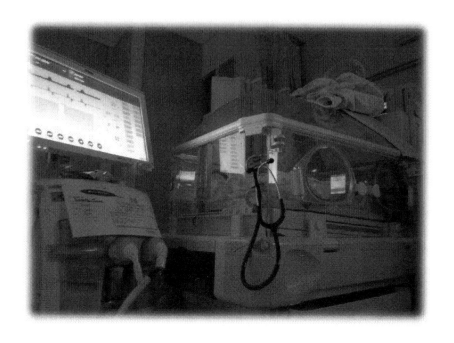

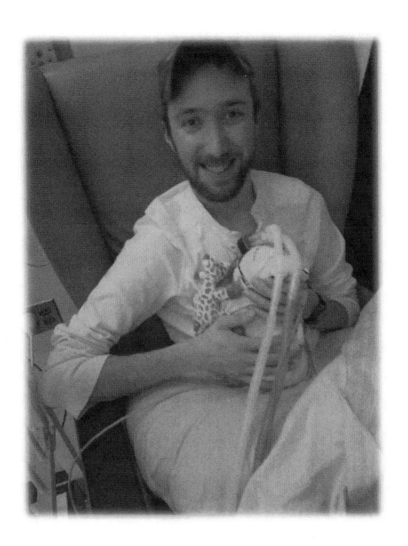

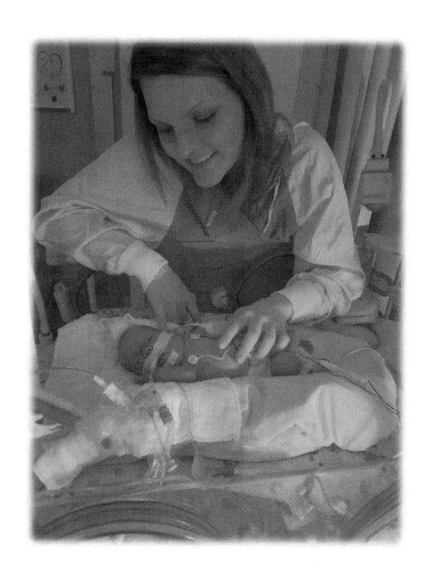

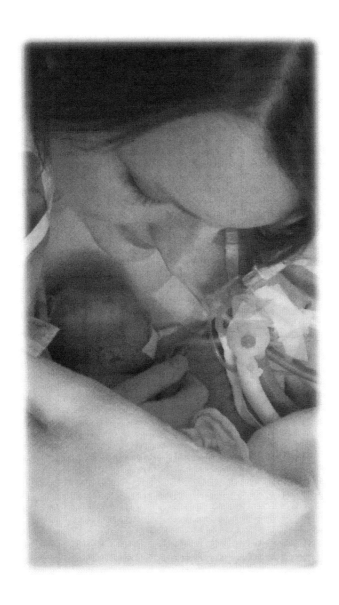

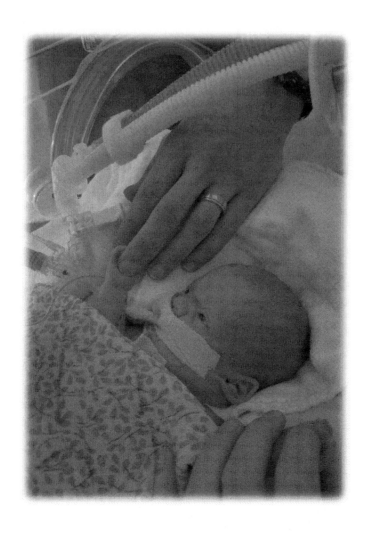

Discharge Day- 01/24/2018
136 NICU Days

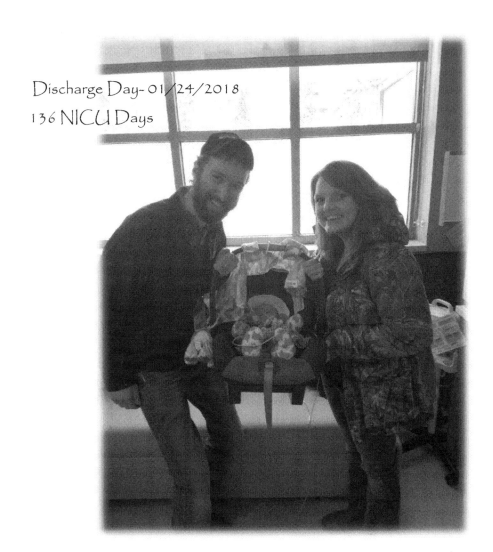

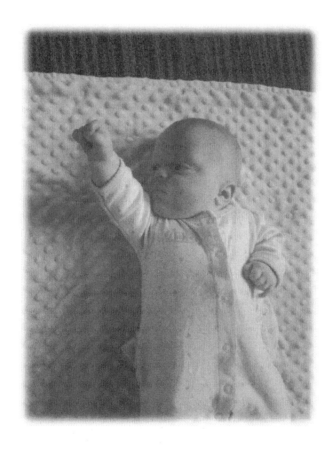